Locked In Reflection

Locked In Reflection

Matthew Petchinsky

Locked In Reflection: A Chastity Journey Through Locktober
By: Matthew Petchinsky

Introduction to "Locked In Reflection: A Chastity Journey Through Locktober"

Hello Kinksters! Happy Locktober!

Welcome to an exciting and empowering month dedicated to exploring the depths of control, restraint, and self-discipline. Locktober isn't just about physical chastity—it's about mental and emotional growth, building resilience, and pushing your limits in the most personal and intimate ways. Whether this is your first Locktober or you're a seasoned veteran, this journal will guide you through each day, helping you reflect on your experiences and learn more about yourself.

"Locked In Reflection" is not just a place to record your journey; it's a tool for self-discovery. Through daily entries, weekly reviews, and a final monthly reflection, you'll have the opportunity to dive deep into your thoughts, emotions, and progress. You'll track not only your successes but also your challenges, uncovering new layers of yourself as you navigate through this exhilarating experience.

Throughout Locktober, you may encounter moments of temptation, frustration, or even triumph. Each of these moments is a powerful opportunity for growth, and this journal is designed to capture them all. It's here to support you, offering prompts that help you stay focused and reflect on your experiences with honesty and intention.

Whether you're participating solo or with a partner, this month is about more than just being locked—it's about exploring what chastity means for you, how it affects your relationships, and what it teaches you about control, desire, and fulfillment.

So, get ready to embark on this transformative journey. May you find strength in restraint, pleasure in patience, and wisdom in reflection.

Let's make this Locktober the best one yet! Happy locking, and happy reflecting!

My Keyholder is:_________________________
Release Date_____________________________

Day 1:
Daily Entry
Date:
Day of Locktober: (e.g., Day 1, Day 15, etc.)

Physical Status:
Any discomfort?

Describe any physical sensations (tightness, pressure, or relaxation).

Was there any need for adjustments today?

Mental State:
How are you feeling emotionally today?

Did you experience any frustration, excitement, calmness, or other emotions?

Challenges:
Did anything test your willpower or commitment today?

How did you manage these challenges? Any close calls or temptations?

Partner Interaction (if applicable):
Did your partner play a role today (teasing, controlling, encouragement)?

Describe any notable experiences or conversations with them.

Activities:
What activities did you do to keep distracted or focused today?

Did you engage in any self-care practices?

Reflections:

What did you learn about yourself today?

Any insights or thoughts on chastity and control?

Affirmations:

Write a short affirmation to motivate yourself (e.g., "I am in control of my desires.").

Day 2:
Daily Entry
Date:
Day of Locktober: (e.g., Day 1, Day 15, etc.)

Physical Status:
Any discomfort?

Describe any physical sensations (tightness, pressure, or relaxation).

Was there any need for adjustments today?

Mental State:

How are you feeling emotionally today?

Did you experience any frustration, excitement, calmness, or other emotions?

Challenges:
Did anything test your willpower or commitment today?

How did you manage these challenges? Any close calls or temptations?

Partner Interaction (if applicable):
Did your partner play a role today (teasing, controlling, encouragement)?

Describe any notable experiences or conversations with them.

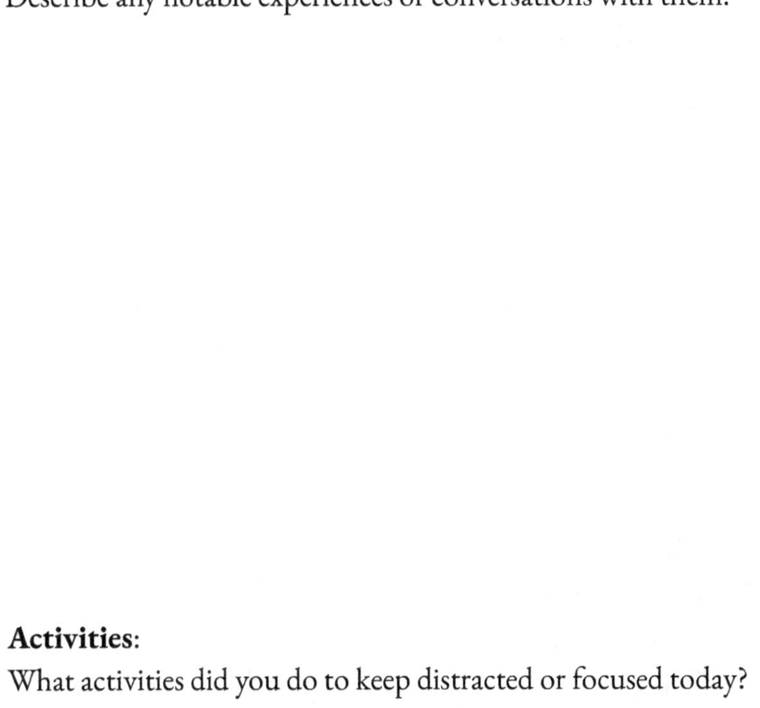

Activities:

What activities did you do to keep distracted or focused today?

Did you engage in any self-care practices?

Reflections:
What did you learn about yourself today?

Any insights or thoughts on chastity and control?

Affirmations:
Write a short affirmation to motivate yourself (e.g., "I am in control of my desires.").

Day 3:
Daily Entry
Date:
Day of Locktober: (e.g., Day 1, Day 15, etc.)

Physical Status:
Any discomfort?

Describe any physical sensations (tightness, pressure, or relaxation).

Was there any need for adjustments today?

Mental State:
How are you feeling emotionally today?

Did you experience any frustration, excitement, calmness, or other emotions?

Challenges:
Did anything test your willpower or commitment today?

How did you manage these challenges? Any close calls or temptations?

Partner Interaction (if applicable):
Did your partner play a role today (teasing, controlling, encourage-ment)?

Describe any notable experiences or conversations with them.

Activities:
What activities did you do to keep distracted or focused today?

Did you engage in any self-care practices?

Reflections:
What did you learn about yourself today?

Any insights or thoughts on chastity and control?

Affirmations:

Write a short affirmation to motivate yourself (e.g., "I am in control of my desires.").

Day 4:
Daily Entry
Date:
Day of Locktober: (e.g., Day 1, Day 15, etc.)

Physical Status:
Any discomfort?

Describe any physical sensations (tightness, pressure, or relaxation).

Was there any need for adjustments today?

Mental State:

How are you feeling emotionally today?

Did you experience any frustration, excitement, calmness, or other emotions?

Challenges:

Did anything test your willpower or commitment today?

How did you manage these challenges? Any close calls or temptations?

Partner Interaction (if applicable):
Did your partner play a role today (teasing, controlling, encouragement)?

Describe any notable experiences or conversations with them.

Activities:

What activities did you do to keep distracted or focused today?

Did you engage in any self-care practices?

Reflections:

What did you learn about yourself today?

Any insights or thoughts on chastity and control?

Affirmations:
Write a short affirmation to motivate yourself (e.g., "I am in control of my desires.").

Day 5:
Daily Entry
Date:
Day of Locktober: (e.g., Day 1, Day 15, etc.)

Physical Status:
Any discomfort?

Describe any physical sensations (tightness, pressure, or relaxation).

Was there any need for adjustments today?

Mental State:
How are you feeling emotionally today?

Did you experience any frustration, excitement, calmness, or other emotions?

Challenges:
Did anything test your willpower or commitment today?

How did you manage these challenges? Any close calls or temptations?

Partner Interaction (if applicable):
Did your partner play a role today (teasing, controlling, encouragement)?

Describe any notable experiences or conversations with them.

Activities:

What activities did you do to keep distracted or focused today?

Did you engage in any self-care practices?

Reflections:

What did you learn about yourself today?

Any insights or thoughts on chastity and control?

Affirmations:

Write a short affirmation to motivate yourself (e.g., "I am in control of my desires.").

Day 6:
Daily Entry
Date:
Day of Locktober: (e.g., Day 1, Day 15, etc.)

Physical Status:
Any discomfort?

Describe any physical sensations (tightness, pressure, or relaxation).

Was there any need for adjustments today?

Mental State:

How are you feeling emotionally today?

Did you experience any frustration, excitement, calmness, or other emotions?

Challenges:
Did anything test your willpower or commitment today?

How did you manage these challenges? Any close calls or temptations?

Partner Interaction (if applicable):
Did your partner play a role today (teasing, controlling, encouragement)?

Describe any notable experiences or conversations with them.

Activities:
What activities did you do to keep distracted or focused today?

Did you engage in any self-care practices?

Reflections:
What did you learn about yourself today?

Any insights or thoughts on chastity and control?

Affirmations:

Write a short affirmation to motivate yourself (e.g., "I am in control of my desires.").

Day 7:
Daily Entry
Date:
Day of Locktober: (e.g., Day 1, Day 15, etc.)

Physical Status:
Any discomfort?

Describe any physical sensations (tightness, pressure, or relaxation).

Was there any need for adjustments today?

Mental State:

How are you feeling emotionally today?

Did you experience any frustration, excitement, calmness, or other emotions?

Challenges:

Did anything test your willpower or commitment today?

How did you manage these challenges? Any close calls or temptations?

Partner Interaction (if applicable):

Did your partner play a role today (teasing, controlling, encouragement)?

Describe any notable experiences or conversations with them.

Activities:

What activities did you do to keep distracted or focused today?

Did you engage in any self-care practices?

Reflections:

What did you learn about yourself today?

Any insights or thoughts on chastity and control?

Affirmations:

Write a short affirmation to motivate yourself (e.g., "I am in control of my desires.").

<u>Week 1 Review:</u>
Weekly Review
Week Number: (Week 1, Week 2, etc.)

Overall Feelings:
How do you feel after completing another week?

Are you noticing any shifts in your mental or emotional state?

Progress:
How successful were you in staying locked?

Did you meet your goals for the week?

Physical Changes:
Are there any changes to your physical comfort level?

Have you adapted to the chastity device in any way?

Emotional Challenges:
What emotional hurdles did you encounter this week?

How did you overcome or cope with them?

Partner Dynamic:
Has your relationship or interaction with your partner evolved this week?

How has chastity influenced your connection?

Key Takeaways:
What were the most significant lessons or insights from the week?

Any strategies for the coming week?

Goals for Next Week:
List your goals or intentions for the next week.

Day 8:
Daily Entry
Date:
Day of Locktober: (e.g., Day 1, Day 15, etc.)

Physical Status:
Any discomfort?

Describe any physical sensations (tightness, pressure, or relaxation).

Was there any need for adjustments today?

Mental State:

How are you feeling emotionally today?

Did you experience any frustration, excitement, calmness, or other emotions?

Challenges:
Did anything test your willpower or commitment today?

How did you manage these challenges? Any close calls or temptations?

Partner Interaction (if applicable):
Did your partner play a role today (teasing, controlling, encouragement)?

Describe any notable experiences or conversations with them.

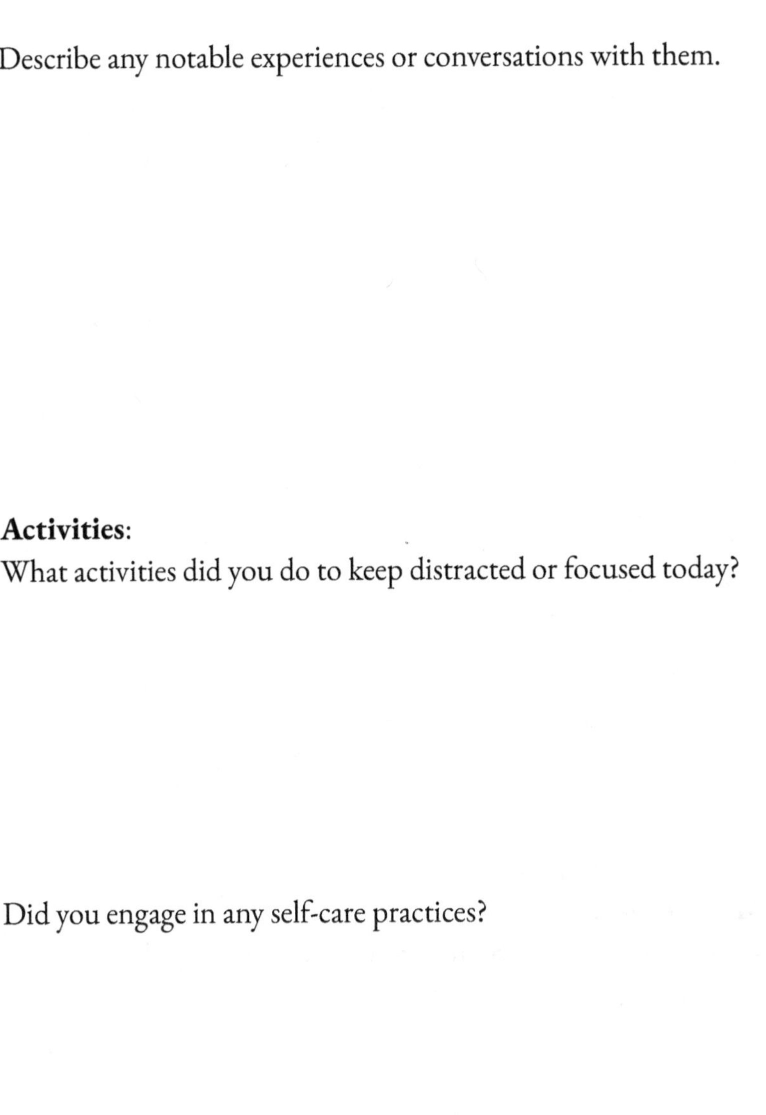

Activities:
What activities did you do to keep distracted or focused today?

Did you engage in any self-care practices?

Reflections:
What did you learn about yourself today?

Any insights or thoughts on chastity and control?

Affirmations:
Write a short affirmation to motivate yourself (e.g., "I am in control of my desires.").

Day 9:
Daily Entry
Date:
Day of Locktober: (e.g., Day 1, Day 15, etc.)

Physical Status:
Any discomfort?

Describe any physical sensations (tightness, pressure, or relaxation).

Was there any need for adjustments today?

Mental State:
How are you feeling emotionally today?

Did you experience any frustration, excitement, calmness, or other emotions?

Challenges:
Did anything test your willpower or commitment today?

How did you manage these challenges? Any close calls or temptations?

Partner Interaction (if applicable):
Did your partner play a role today (teasing, controlling, encouragement)?

Describe any notable experiences or conversations with them.

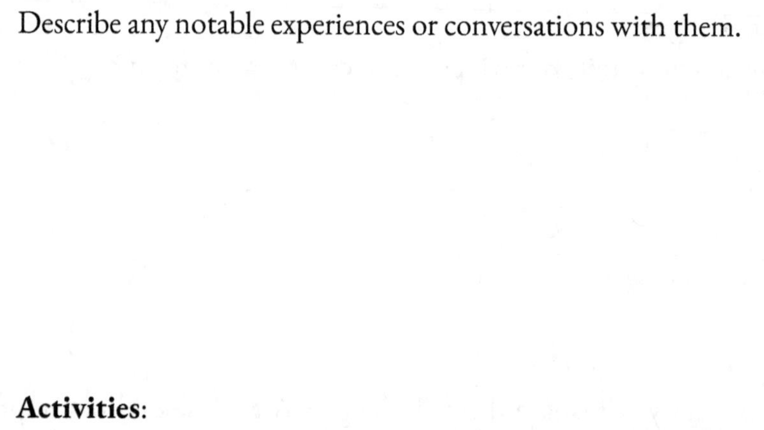

Activities:
What activities did you do to keep distracted or focused today?

Did you engage in any self-care practices?

Reflections:
What did you learn about yourself today?

Any insights or thoughts on chastity and control?

Affirmations:
Write a short affirmation to motivate yourself (e.g., "I am in control of my desires.").

Day 10:
Daily Entry
Date:
Day of Locktober: (e.g., Day 1, Day 15, etc.)

Physical Status:
Any discomfort?

Describe any physical sensations (tightness, pressure, or relaxation).

Was there any need for adjustments today?

Mental State:

How are you feeling emotionally today?

Did you experience any frustration, excitement, calmness, or other emotions?

Challenges:

Did anything test your willpower or commitment today?

How did you manage these challenges? Any close calls or temptations?

Partner Interaction (if applicable):
Did your partner play a role today (teasing, controlling, encouragement)?

Describe any notable experiences or conversations with them.

Activities:
What activities did you do to keep distracted or focused today?

Did you engage in any self-care practices?

Reflections:
What did you learn about yourself today?

Any insights or thoughts on chastity and control?

Affirmations:
Write a short affirmation to motivate yourself (e.g., "I am in control of my desires.").

Day 11:
Daily Entry
Date:
Day of Locktober: (e.g., Day 1, Day 15, etc.)

Physical Status:
Any discomfort?

Describe any physical sensations (tightness, pressure, or relaxation).

Was there any need for adjustments today?

Mental State:
How are you feeling emotionally today?

Did you experience any frustration, excitement, calmness, or other emotions?

Challenges:
Did anything test your willpower or commitment today?

How did you manage these challenges? Any close calls or temptations?

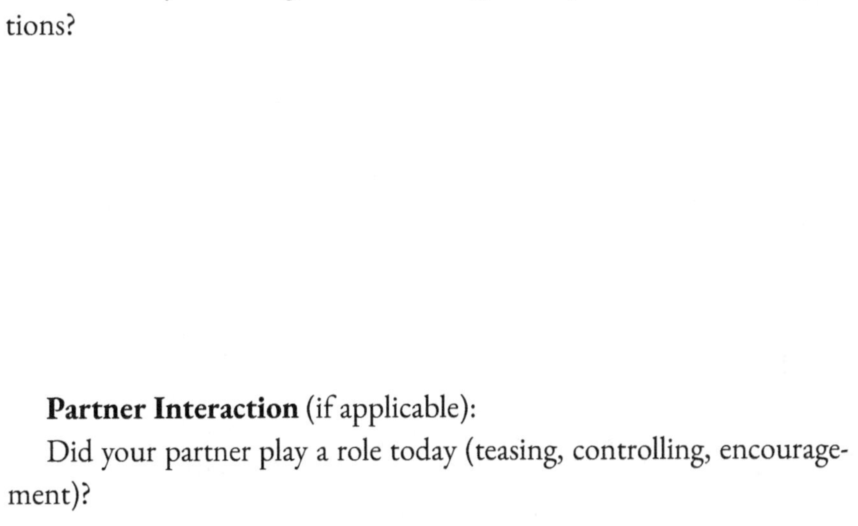

Partner Interaction (if applicable):
Did your partner play a role today (teasing, controlling, encouragement)?

Describe any notable experiences or conversations with them.

Activities:
What activities did you do to keep distracted or focused today?

Did you engage in any self-care practices?

Reflections:
What did you learn about yourself today?

Any insights or thoughts on chastity and control?

Affirmations:
Write a short affirmation to motivate yourself (e.g., "I am in control of my desires.").

Day 12:
Daily Entry
Date:
Day of Locktober: (e.g., Day 1, Day 15, etc.)

Physical Status:
Any discomfort?

Describe any physical sensations (tightness, pressure, or relaxation).

Was there any need for adjustments today?

Mental State:
How are you feeling emotionally today?

Did you experience any frustration, excitement, calmness, or other emotions?

Challenges:
Did anything test your willpower or commitment today?

How did you manage these challenges? Any close calls or temptations?

Partner Interaction (if applicable):
Did your partner play a role today (teasing, controlling, encouragement)?

Describe any notable experiences or conversations with them.

Activities:

What activities did you do to keep distracted or focused today?

Did you engage in any self-care practices?

Reflections:

What did you learn about yourself today?

Any insights or thoughts on chastity and control?

Affirmations:

Write a short affirmation to motivate yourself (e.g., "I am in control of my desires.").

Day 13:
Daily Entry
Date:
Day of Locktober: (e.g., Day 1, Day 15, etc.)

Physical Status:
Any discomfort?

Describe any physical sensations (tightness, pressure, or relaxation).

Was there any need for adjustments today?

Mental State:
How are you feeling emotionally today?

Did you experience any frustration, excitement, calmness, or other emotions?

Challenges:
Did anything test your willpower or commitment today?

How did you manage these challenges? Any close calls or temptations?

Partner Interaction (if applicable):
Did your partner play a role today (teasing, controlling, encouragement)?

Describe any notable experiences or conversations with them.

Activities:

What activities did you do to keep distracted or focused today?

Did you engage in any self-care practices?

Reflections:
What did you learn about yourself today?

Any insights or thoughts on chastity and control?

Affirmations:
Write a short affirmation to motivate yourself (e.g., "I am in control of my desires.").

Day 14:
Daily Entry
Date:
Day of Locktober: (e.g., Day 1, Day 15, etc.)

Physical Status:
Any discomfort?

Describe any physical sensations (tightness, pressure, or relaxation).

Was there any need for adjustments today?

Mental State:
How are you feeling emotionally today?

Did you experience any frustration, excitement, calmness, or other emotions?

Challenges:
Did anything test your willpower or commitment today?

How did you manage these challenges? Any close calls or temptations?

Partner Interaction (if applicable):
Did your partner play a role today (teasing, controlling, encouragement)?

Describe any notable experiences or conversations with them.

Activities:

What activities did you do to keep distracted or focused today?

Did you engage in any self-care practices?

Reflections:

What did you learn about yourself today?

Any insights or thoughts on chastity and control?

Affirmations:

Write a short affirmation to motivate yourself (e.g., "I am in control of my desires.").

<u>**Week 2 Review:**</u>
Weekly Review
Week Number: (Week 1, Week 2, etc.)

Overall Feelings:
How do you feel after completing another week?

Are you noticing any shifts in your mental or emotional state?

Progress:
How successful were you in staying locked?

Did you meet your goals for the week?

Physical Changes:
Are there any changes to your physical comfort level?

Have you adapted to the chastity device in any way?

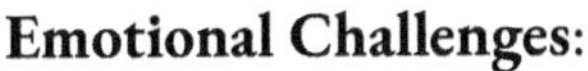

Emotional Challenges:
What emotional hurdles did you encounter this week?

How did you overcome or cope with them?

Partner Dynamic:
Has your relationship or interaction with your partner evolved this week?

How has chastity influenced your connection?

Key Takeaways:
What were the most significant lessons or insights from the week?

Any strategies for the coming week?

Goals for Next Week:
List your goals or intentions for the next week.

Day 15:
Daily Entry
Date:
Day of Locktober: (e.g., Day 1, Day 15, etc.)

Physical Status:
Any discomfort?

Describe any physical sensations (tightness, pressure, or relaxation).

Was there any need for adjustments today?

Mental State:

How are you feeling emotionally today?

Did you experience any frustration, excitement, calmness, or other emotions?

Challenges:
Did anything test your willpower or commitment today?

How did you manage these challenges? Any close calls or temptations?

Partner Interaction (if applicable):
Did your partner play a role today (teasing, controlling, encouragement)?

Describe any notable experiences or conversations with them.

Activities:

What activities did you do to keep distracted or focused today?

Did you engage in any self-care practices?

Reflections:
What did you learn about yourself today?

Any insights or thoughts on chastity and control?

Affirmations:
Write a short affirmation to motivate yourself (e.g., "I am in control of my desires.").

Day 16:
Daily Entry
Date:
Day of Locktober: (e.g., Day 1, Day 15, etc.)

Physical Status:
Any discomfort?

Describe any physical sensations (tightness, pressure, or relaxation).

Was there any need for adjustments today?

Mental State:

How are you feeling emotionally today?

Did you experience any frustration, excitement, calmness, or other emotions?

Challenges:

Did anything test your willpower or commitment today?

How did you manage these challenges? Any close calls or temptations?

Partner Interaction (if applicable):
Did your partner play a role today (teasing, controlling, encouragement)?

Describe any notable experiences or conversations with them.

Activities:

What activities did you do to keep distracted or focused today?

Did you engage in any self-care practices?

Reflections:

What did you learn about yourself today?

Any insights or thoughts on chastity and control?

Affirmations:

Write a short affirmation to motivate yourself (e.g., "I am in control of my desires.").

Day 17:
Daily Entry
Date:
Day of Locktober: (e.g., Day 1, Day 15, etc.)

Physical Status:
Any discomfort?

Describe any physical sensations (tightness, pressure, or relaxation).

Was there any need for adjustments today?

Mental State:
How are you feeling emotionally today?

Did you experience any frustration, excitement, calmness, or other emotions?

Challenges:
Did anything test your willpower or commitment today?

How did you manage these challenges? Any close calls or temptations?

Partner Interaction (if applicable):
Did your partner play a role today (teasing, controlling, encouragement)?

Describe any notable experiences or conversations with them.

Activities:

What activities did you do to keep distracted or focused today?

Did you engage in any self-care practices?

Reflections:

What did you learn about yourself today?

Any insights or thoughts on chastity and control?

Affirmations:

Write a short affirmation to motivate yourself (e.g., "I am in control of my desires.").

Day 18:
Daily Entry
Date:
Day of Locktober: (e.g., Day 1, Day 15, etc.)

Physical Status:
Any discomfort?

Describe any physical sensations (tightness, pressure, or relaxation).

Was there any need for adjustments today?

Mental State:
How are you feeling emotionally today?

Did you experience any frustration, excitement, calmness, or other emotions?

Challenges:
Did anything test your willpower or commitment today?

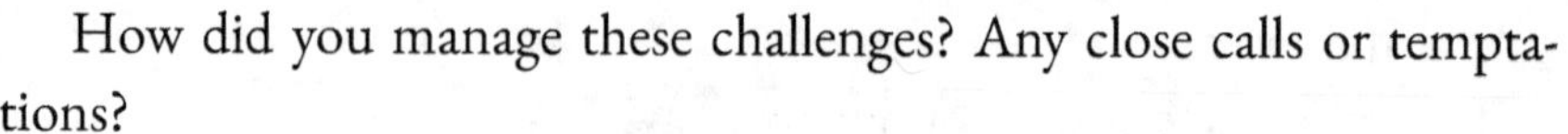

How did you manage these challenges? Any close calls or temptations?

Partner Interaction (if applicable):
Did your partner play a role today (teasing, controlling, encouragement)?

Describe any notable experiences or conversations with them.

Activities:
What activities did you do to keep distracted or focused today?

Did you engage in any self-care practices?

Reflections:
What did you learn about yourself today?

Any insights or thoughts on chastity and control?

Affirmations:

Write a short affirmation to motivate yourself (e.g., "I am in control of my desires.").

Day 19:
Daily Entry
Date:
Day of Locktober: (e.g., Day 1, Day 15, etc.)

Physical Status:
Any discomfort?

Describe any physical sensations (tightness, pressure, or relaxation).

Was there any need for adjustments today?

Mental State:
How are you feeling emotionally today?

Did you experience any frustration, excitement, calmness, or other emotions?

Challenges:
Did anything test your willpower or commitment today?

How did you manage these challenges? Any close calls or temptations?

Partner Interaction (if applicable):
Did your partner play a role today (teasing, controlling, encouragement)?

Describe any notable experiences or conversations with them.

Activities:
What activities did you do to keep distracted or focused today?

Did you engage in any self-care practices?

Reflections:
What did you learn about yourself today?

Any insights or thoughts on chastity and control?

Affirmations:

Write a short affirmation to motivate yourself (e.g., "I am in control of my desires.").

Day 20:
Daily Entry
Date:
Day of Locktober: (e.g., Day 1, Day 15, etc.)

Physical Status:
Any discomfort?

Describe any physical sensations (tightness, pressure, or relaxation).

Was there any need for adjustments today?

Mental State:
How are you feeling emotionally today?

Did you experience any frustration, excitement, calmness, or other emotions?

Challenges:
Did anything test your willpower or commitment today?

How did you manage these challenges? Any close calls or tempta-tions?

Partner Interaction (if applicable):

Did your partner play a role today (teasing, controlling, encourage-ment)?

Describe any notable experiences or conversations with them.

Activities:
What activities did you do to keep distracted or focused today?

Did you engage in any self-care practices?

Reflections:
What did you learn about yourself today?

Any insights or thoughts on chastity and control?

Affirmations:

Write a short affirmation to motivate yourself (e.g., "I am in control of my desires.").

Day 21:
Daily Entry
Date:
Day of Locktober: (e.g., Day 1, Day 15, etc.)

Physical Status:
Any discomfort?

Describe any physical sensations (tightness, pressure, or relaxation).

Was there any need for adjustments today?

Mental State:
How are you feeling emotionally today?

Did you experience any frustration, excitement, calmness, or other emotions?

Challenges:
Did anything test your willpower or commitment today?

How did you manage these challenges? Any close calls or temptations?

Partner Interaction (if applicable):
Did your partner play a role today (teasing, controlling, encouragement)?

Describe any notable experiences or conversations with them.

Activities:

What activities did you do to keep distracted or focused today?

Did you engage in any self-care practices?

Reflections:
What did you learn about yourself today?

Any insights or thoughts on chastity and control?

Affirmations:
Write a short affirmation to motivate yourself (e.g., "I am in control of my desires.").

<u>**Week 3 Review:**</u>
Weekly Review
Week Number: (Week 1, Week 2, etc.)

Overall Feelings:
How do you feel after completing another week?

Are you noticing any shifts in your mental or emotional state?

Progress:
How successful were you in staying locked?

Did you meet your goals for the week?

Physical Changes:
Are there any changes to your physical comfort level?

Have you adapted to the chastity device in any way?

Emotional Challenges:
What emotional hurdles did you encounter this week?

How did you overcome or cope with them?

Partner Dynamic:

Has your relationship or interaction with your partner evolved this week?

How has chastity influenced your connection?

Key Takeaways:
What were the most significant lessons or insights from the week?

Any strategies for the coming week?

Goals for Next Week:
List your goals or intentions for the next week.

Day 22:
Daily Entry
Date:
Day of Locktober: (e.g., Day 1, Day 15, etc.)

Physical Status:
Any discomfort?

Describe any physical sensations (tightness, pressure, or relaxation).

Was there any need for adjustments today?

Mental State:
How are you feeling emotionally today?

Did you experience any frustration, excitement, calmness, or other emotions?

Challenges:
Did anything test your willpower or commitment today?

How did you manage these challenges? Any close calls or temptations?

Partner Interaction (if applicable):
Did your partner play a role today (teasing, controlling, encouragement)?

Describe any notable experiences or conversations with them.

Activities:

What activities did you do to keep distracted or focused today?

Did you engage in any self-care practices?

Reflections:

What did you learn about yourself today?

Any insights or thoughts on chastity and control?

Affirmations:
Write a short affirmation to motivate yourself (e.g., "I am in control of my desires.").

Day 23:
Daily Entry
Date:
Day of Locktober: (e.g., Day 1, Day 15, etc.)

Physical Status:
Any discomfort?

Describe any physical sensations (tightness, pressure, or relaxation).

Was there any need for adjustments today?

Mental State:
How are you feeling emotionally today?

Did you experience any frustration, excitement, calmness, or other emotions?

Challenges:
Did anything test your willpower or commitment today?

How did you manage these challenges? Any close calls or temptations?

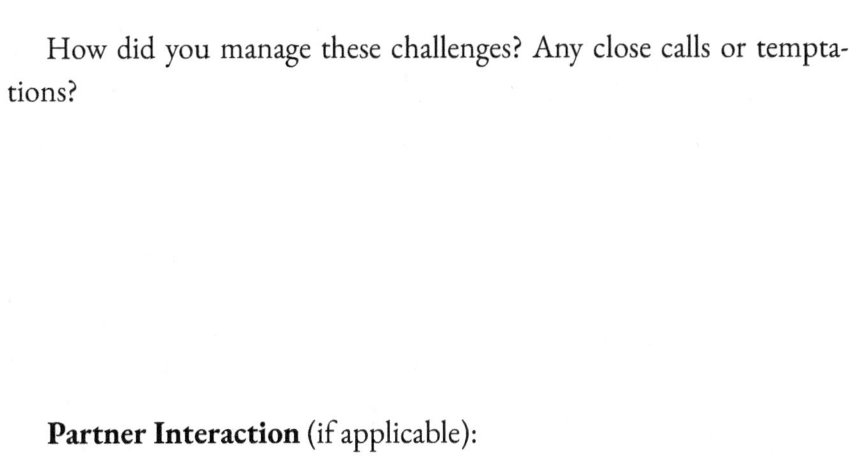

Partner Interaction (if applicable):
Did your partner play a role today (teasing, controlling, encouragement)?

Describe any notable experiences or conversations with them.

Activities:

What activities did you do to keep distracted or focused today?

Did you engage in any self-care practices?

Reflections:

What did you learn about yourself today?

Any insights or thoughts on chastity and control?

Affirmations:

Write a short affirmation to motivate yourself (e.g., "I am in control of my desires.").

Day 24:
Daily Entry
Date:
Day of Locktober: (e.g., Day 1, Day 15, etc.)

Physical Status:
Any discomfort?

Describe any physical sensations (tightness, pressure, or relaxation).

Was there any need for adjustments today?

Mental State:

How are you feeling emotionally today?

Did you experience any frustration, excitement, calmness, or other emotions?

Challenges:
Did anything test your willpower or commitment today?

How did you manage these challenges? Any close calls or temptations?

Partner Interaction (if applicable):

Did your partner play a role today (teasing, controlling, encourage-ment)?

Describe any notable experiences or conversations with them.

Activities:
What activities did you do to keep distracted or focused today?

Did you engage in any self-care practices?

Reflections:
What did you learn about yourself today?

Any insights or thoughts on chastity and control?

Affirmations:

Write a short affirmation to motivate yourself (e.g., "I am in control of my desires.").

Day 25:
Daily Entry
Date:
Day of Locktober: (e.g., Day 1, Day 15, etc.)

Physical Status:
Any discomfort?

Describe any physical sensations (tightness, pressure, or relaxation).

Was there any need for adjustments today?

Mental State:
How are you feeling emotionally today?

Did you experience any frustration, excitement, calmness, or other emotions?

Challenges:
Did anything test your willpower or commitment today?

How did you manage these challenges? Any close calls or tempta-tions?

Partner Interaction (if applicable):
Did your partner play a role today (teasing, controlling, encourage-ment)?

Describe any notable experiences or conversations with them.

Activities:
What activities did you do to keep distracted or focused today?

Did you engage in any self-care practices?

Reflections:
What did you learn about yourself today?

Any insights or thoughts on chastity and control?

Affirmations:

Write a short affirmation to motivate yourself (e.g., "I am in control of my desires.").

Day 26:
Daily Entry
Date:
Day of Locktober: (e.g., Day 1, Day 15, etc.)

Physical Status:
Any discomfort?

Describe any physical sensations (tightness, pressure, or relaxation).

Was there any need for adjustments today?

Mental State:
How are you feeling emotionally today?

Did you experience any frustration, excitement, calmness, or other emotions?

Challenges:
Did anything test your willpower or commitment today?

How did you manage these challenges? Any close calls or temptations?

Partner Interaction (if applicable):
Did your partner play a role today (teasing, controlling, encouragement)?

Describe any notable experiences or conversations with them.

Activities:

What activities did you do to keep distracted or focused today?

Did you engage in any self-care practices?

Reflections:
What did you learn about yourself today?

Any insights or thoughts on chastity and control?

Affirmations:
Write a short affirmation to motivate yourself (e.g., "I am in control of my desires.").

Day 27:
Daily Entry
Date:
Day of Locktober: (e.g., Day 1, Day 15, etc.)

Physical Status:
Any discomfort?

Describe any physical sensations (tightness, pressure, or relaxation).

Was there any need for adjustments today?

Mental State:
How are you feeling emotionally today?

Did you experience any frustration, excitement, calmness, or other emotions?

Challenges:
Did anything test your willpower or commitment today?

How did you manage these challenges? Any close calls or temptations?

Partner Interaction (if applicable):
Did your partner play a role today (teasing, controlling, encouragement)?

Describe any notable experiences or conversations with them.

Activities:

What activities did you do to keep distracted or focused today?

Did you engage in any self-care practices?

Reflections:
What did you learn about yourself today?

Any insights or thoughts on chastity and control?

Affirmations:
Write a short affirmation to motivate yourself (e.g., "I am in control of my desires.").

Day 28:
Daily Entry
Date:
Day of Locktober: (e.g., Day 1, Day 15, etc.)

Physical Status:
Any discomfort?

Describe any physical sensations (tightness, pressure, or relaxation).

Was there any need for adjustments today?

Mental State:

How are you feeling emotionally today?

Did you experience any frustration, excitement, calmness, or other emotions?

Challenges:
Did anything test your willpower or commitment today?

How did you manage these challenges? Any close calls or temptations?

Partner Interaction (if applicable):
Did your partner play a role today (teasing, controlling, encouragement)?

Describe any notable experiences or conversations with them.

Activities:

What activities did you do to keep distracted or focused today?

Did you engage in any self-care practices?

Reflections:
What did you learn about yourself today?

Any insights or thoughts on chastity and control?

Affirmations:
Write a short affirmation to motivate yourself (e.g., "I am in control of my desires.").

<u>**Week 4 Review:**</u>
Weekly Review
Week Number: (Week 1, Week 2, etc.)

Overall Feelings:
How do you feel after completing another week?

Are you noticing any shifts in your mental or emotional state?

Progress:
How successful were you in staying locked?

Did you meet your goals for the week?

Physical Changes:
Are there any changes to your physical comfort level?

Have you adapted to the chastity device in any way?

Emotional Challenges:
What emotional hurdles did you encounter this week?

How did you overcome or cope with them?

Partner Dynamic:

Has your relationship or interaction with your partner evolved this week?

How has chastity influenced your connection?

Key Takeaways:
What were the most significant lessons or insights from the week?

Any strategies for the coming week?

Goals for Next Week:

List your goals or intentions for the next week.

Day 29:
Daily Entry
Date:
Day of Locktober: (e.g., Day 1, Day 15, etc.)

Physical Status:
Any discomfort?

Describe any physical sensations (tightness, pressure, or relaxation).

Was there any need for adjustments today?

Mental State:

How are you feeling emotionally today?

Did you experience any frustration, excitement, calmness, or other emotions?

Challenges:
Did anything test your willpower or commitment today?

How did you manage these challenges? Any close calls or temptations?

Partner Interaction (if applicable):
Did your partner play a role today (teasing, controlling, encouragement)?

Describe any notable experiences or conversations with them.

Activities:
What activities did you do to keep distracted or focused today?

Did you engage in any self-care practices?

Reflections:
What did you learn about yourself today?

Any insights or thoughts on chastity and control?

Affirmations:
Write a short affirmation to motivate yourself (e.g., "I am in control of my desires.").

Day 30:
Daily Entry
Date:
Day of Locktober: (e.g., Day 1, Day 15, etc.)

Physical Status:
Any discomfort?

Describe any physical sensations (tightness, pressure, or relaxation).

Was there any need for adjustments today?

Mental State:
How are you feeling emotionally today?

Did you experience any frustration, excitement, calmness, or other emotions?

Challenges:
Did anything test your willpower or commitment today?

How did you manage these challenges? Any close calls or temptations?

Partner Interaction (if applicable):
Did your partner play a role today (teasing, controlling, encouragement)?

Describe any notable experiences or conversations with them.

Activities:

What activities did you do to keep distracted or focused today?

Did you engage in any self-care practices?

Reflections:
What did you learn about yourself today?

Any insights or thoughts on chastity and control?

Affirmations:
Write a short affirmation to motivate yourself (e.g., "I am in control of my desires.").

Day 31:
Daily Entry
Date:
Day of Locktober: (e.g., Day 1, Day 15, etc.)

Physical Status:
Any discomfort?

Describe any physical sensations (tightness, pressure, or relaxation).

Was there any need for adjustments today?

Mental State:
How are you feeling emotionally today?

Did you experience any frustration, excitement, calmness, or other emotions?

Challenges:
Did anything test your willpower or commitment today?

How did you manage these challenges? Any close calls or temptations?

Partner Interaction (if applicable):
Did your partner play a role today (teasing, controlling, encouragement)?

Describe any notable experiences or conversations with them.

Activities:
What activities did you do to keep distracted or focused today?

Did you engage in any self-care practices?

Reflections:
What did you learn about yourself today?

Any insights or thoughts on chastity and control?

Affirmations:
Write a short affirmation to motivate yourself (e.g., "I am in control of my desires.").

Monthly Review
Final Thoughts on Locktober:
How do you feel at the end of the month compared to the beginning?

Major Lessons Learned:
What were the most important lessons you've gained throughout Locktober?

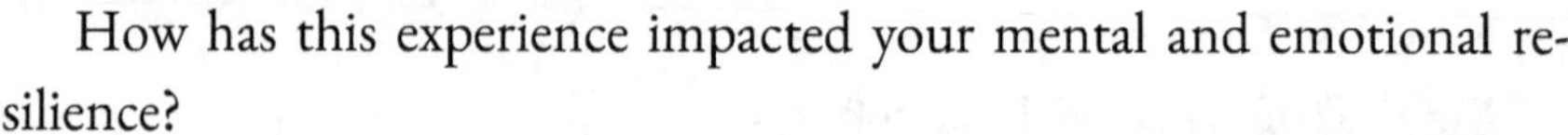

Emotional and Mental Growth:
How has this experience impacted your mental and emotional resilience?

Have you noticed personal growth in any area of your life?

Physical Condition:
Reflect on any physical changes, improvements, or issues from the chastity challenge.

Challenges and Triumphs:
What were the hardest parts of the journey, and how did you overcome them?

What were your biggest victories?

Partner Connection:
Reflect on how your relationship with your partner has changed (if applicable).

Has the power dynamic or emotional intimacy shifted?

Personal Empowerment:
How has chastity changed your view on control, power, and self-discipline?

Future Plans:
Will you continue with chastity after Locktober ends?

What goals will you set for your next challenge?

Conclusion: Thank You and Stay Safe

As Locktober comes to a close, we want to take a moment to thank you for embarking on this journey with "Locked In Reflection: A Chastity Journey Through Locktober." Whether this was your first time or you're a seasoned participant, your commitment to self-discipline, introspection, and growth is something to be truly proud of.

By purchasing this journal, you've taken a step toward deepening your understanding of chastity, control, and the power of restraint. We hope that through these pages, you've not only tracked your progress but also uncovered new insights about yourself and your relationships. It's our hope that these reflections continue to guide you long after Locktober has ended.

Remember, Locktober is more than just a physical challenge—it's a mental and emotional journey that helps build resilience, trust, and connection with yourself and others. We encourage you to take everything you've learned and apply it to future experiences, whether you continue with chastity or explore new aspects of yourself.

Thank you for allowing us to be a part of your journey, and we wish you all the best in your future explorations. Stay safe, be mindful, and remember that growth comes in many forms, even through the power of restraint.

Happy unlocking, and we hope to see you next Locktober!

<u>Message from the Author:</u>

I hope you enjoyed this book, I love astrology and knew there was not a book such as this out on the shelf. I love metaphysical items as well. Please check out my other books:

-Life of Government Benefits

-My life of Hell

-My life with Hydrocephalus

-Red Sky

-World Domination:Woman's rule

-World Domination:Woman's Rule 2: The War

-Life and Banishment of Apophis: book 1

-The Kidney Friendly Diet

-The Ultimate Hemp Cookbook

-Creating a Dispensary(legally)

-Cleanliness throughout life: the importance of showering from childhood to adulthood.

-Strong Roots: The Risks of Overcoddling children

-Hemp Horoscopes: Cosmic Insights and Earthly Healing

- Celestial Hemp Navigating the Zodiac: Through the Green Cosmos

-Astrological Hemp: Aligning The Stars with Earth's Ancient Herb

-The Astrological Guide to Hemp: Stars, Signs, and Sacred Leaves

-Green Growth: Innovative Marketing Strategies for your Hemp Products and Dispensary

-Cosmic Cannabis

-Astrological Munchies

-Henry The Hemp

-Zodiacal Roots: The Astrological Soul Of Hemp

- **Green Constellations: Intersection of Hemp and Zodiac**

-Hemp in The Houses: An astrological Adventure Through The Cannabis Galaxy

-Galactic Ganja Guide

Heavenly Hemp

Zodiac Leaves
Doctor Who Astrology
Cannastrology
Stellar Satvias and Cosmic Indicas
Celestial Cannabis: A Zodiac Journey
AstroHerbology: The Sky and The Soil: Volume 1
AstroHerbology:Celestial Cannabis:Volume 2
Cosmic Cannabis Cultivation
The Starry Guide to Herbal Harmony: Volume 1
The Starry Guide to Herbal Harmony: Cannabis Universe: Volume 2

Yugioh Astrology: Astrological Guide to Deck, Duels and more
Nightmare Mansion: Echoes of The Abyss
Nightmare Mansion 2: Legacy of Shadows
Nightmare Mansion 3: Shadows of the Forgotten
Nightmare Mansion 4: Echoes of the Damned
The Life and Banishment of Apophis: Book 2
Nightmare Mansion: Halls of Despair
Healing with Herb: Cannabis and Hydrocephalus
Planetary Pot: Aligning with Astrological Herbs: Volume 1
Fast Track to Freedom: 30 Days to Financial Independence Using AI, Assets, and Agile Hustles
Cosmic Hemp Pathways
How to Become Financially Free in 30 Days: 10,000 Paths to Prosperity
Zodiacal Herbage: Astrological Insights: Volume 1
Nightmare Mansion: Whispers in the Walls
The Daleks Invade Atlantis
Henry the hemp and Hydrocephalus

10X The Kidney Friendly Diet
Cannabis Universe: Adult coloring book
Hemp Astrology: The Healing Power of the Stars

Zodiacal Herbage: Astrological Insights: Cannabis Universe: Volume 2

<u>**Planetary Pot: Aligning with Astrological Herbs: Cannabis Universes: Volume 2**</u>

Doctor Who Meets the Replicators and SG-1: The Ultimate Battle for Survival

Nightmare Mansion: Curse of the Blood Moon

<u>**The Celestial Stoner: A Guide to the Zodiac**</u>

Cosmic Pleasures: Sex Toy Astrology for Every Sign

Hydrocephalus Astrology: Navigating the Stars and Healing Waters

Lapis and the Mischievous Chocolate Bar

Celestial Positions: Sexual Astrology for Every Sign

Apophis's Shadow Work Journal: **:** A Journey of Self-Discovery and Healing

Kinky Cosmos: Scxual Kink Astrology for Every Sign

Digital Cosmos: The Astrological Digimon Compendium

Stellar Seeds: The Cosmic Guide to Growing with Astrology

Apophis's Daily Gratitude Journal

Cat Astrology: Feline Mysteries of the Cosmos

The Cosmic Kama Sutra: An Astrological Guide to Sexual Positions

Unleash Your Potential: A Guided Journal Powered by AI Insights

Whispers of the Enchanted Grove

Cosmic Pleasures: An Astrological Guide to Sexual Kinks

369, 12 Manifestation Journal

Whisper of the nocturne journal(blank journal for writing or drawing)

The Boogey Book

If you want solar for your home go here: https://www.harborso-lar.live/apophisenterprises/

Get Some Tarot cards: https://www.makeplayingcards.com/sell/apophis-occult-shop

Get some shirts: https://www.bonfire.com/store/apophis-shirt-emporium/

Instagrams:
@apophis_enterprises,
@apophisbookemporium,
@apophisscardshop
Twitter: @apophisenterpr1 Tiktok:@apophisenterprise
Youtube: @sg1fan23477, @FiresideRetreatKingdom

Podcast: Apophis Chat Zone: https://open.spotify.com/show/
5zXbrCLEV2xzCp8ybrfHsk?si=fb4d4fdbdce44dec

Newsletter: https://apophiss-newsletter-27c897.beehiiv.com/